How to Win the Fertility Battle

Navigating the Path to Parenthood

Jessica W. Brown

Copyright © Jessica W. Brown, 2024.

Disclaimer

The information provided in this book is for general informational purposes only. While every effort has been made to ensure the accuracy of the information contained within this book, the author and publisher assume no responsibility for errors or omissions, or for damages resulting from the use of the information contained herein.

This book is sold with the understanding that the author and publisher are not engaged in rendering legal, financial, medical, or other professional advice. The reader should consult with a professional in the respective field for any such advice.

Table Of Contents

INTRODUCTION

A Success Story: Pregnant After Unexplained Infertility

Mary and Peter's journey to parenthood was distinguished by optimism, resilience, and a pivotal guidebook. They married at 28 and had a few pleasant years together before deciding to create a family. Mary stated, "We wanted to enjoy ourselves first."

When they finally started trying to conceive, they assumed it would happen quickly. However, after several fertile couples have just a 20% probability of conceiving each month.

Determined, she began using an ovulation calendar, while Peter made lifestyle adjustments such as giving up smoking and eating healthier. Despite their attempts, months slipped into years without a pregnancy. The disappointment was intense. Mary felt alone and envious of her friends who conceived easily, while Peter felt helpless and ashamed.

During this challenging time, Mary came across a book called "How to Win the Fertility Battle." She purchased the book and delved into its contents, intrigued and yearning for answers. "It felt like a lifeline," she remarked. The book gave in-depth insights into fertility challenges as well as practical suggestions on the next steps.

Mary and Peter were inspired to see a reproductive specialist after reading the book. The expert performed comprehensive testing but found no clear cause of their infertility, labeling them with unexplained infertility. Initially frustrating, the book had prepared them for this possibility by highlighting the necessity of being proactive and informed.

Their doctor suggested they try intrauterine insemination (IUI) with Clomid, followed by in vitro fertilization (IVF) if necessary. They felt more comfortable navigating these alternatives after reading "How to Win the Fertility Battle" and receiving encouragement. The three IUI cycles were an emotional rollercoaster. Despite their best efforts, Mary did not conceive. The book's chapter on dealing with mental stress was a continuous source of solace. "It made us feel less alone," Mary said.

Encouraged by the book's success stories, they decided to try IVF with preimplantation genetic screening (PGS) to boost their chances. IVF was a difficult procedure that included hormone injections, egg harvesting, and tense waiting. However, the book's advice on having a positive attitude and practical methods for dealing with the treatment was really useful.

Finally, Mary received a call confirming her pregnancy. "It was the happiest day of my life!" she declared. Mary carried her pregnancy to term and gave birth to a healthy child. Peter reflected on their trip and remarked, "All the waiting, all the effort, all the worry was worthwhile to have our son."

Mary and Peter's narrative demonstrates the power of endurance, hope, and accurate information. By following the guidance in "How to Win the Fertility Battle," they overcame infertility and found joy in parenthood.

Infertility can be a challenging and emotionally draining process for couples attempting to conceive. It is characterized as the inability to conceive after 12 months or more of regular, unprotected sexual activity. This issue affects millions of couples globally and can be caused by a variety of circumstances in both men and women.

In this book, I hope to provide a thorough guide to understanding infertility, including diagnostic and treatment choices, as well as emotional support for couples on their fertility journey.

My objective is to provide couples with the knowledge, skills, and resources they need to navigate the complex world of infertility and maximize their chances of having a healthy pregnancy.

Throughout the book, I will explore numerous elements of fertility, such as lifestyle modifications that might boost conception, alternative therapies for fertility enhancement, and the necessity of supporting your partner during this difficult time.

By sharing real-life experiences and success stories, I hope to encourage couples to be positive and resilient as they embark on their journey to parenting.

Finally, my goal is to assist couples in overcoming their fertility challenges and starting the family they have always desired.

CHAPTER 1

Infertility In Men And Women

Male infertility can be caused by a low sperm count or the use of specific drugs. Female infertility can be caused by ovulation abnormalities or endometriosis.

What Is Infertility?

Infertility is described as the inability to conceive after a year of unprotected intercourse. The male partner, the female partner, or both may experience fertility issues. Infertility reduces a person's capacity to have children. It normally does not imply that a person is infertile, or physically incapable of having children.

Many couples experience infertility as a crisis. Fertility issues are frequently associated with feelings of guilt or inadequacy. However, an infertility diagnosis does not necessarily imply sterility. Up to 15% of all couples are infertile, but just 1-2% are sterile. Half of couples who seek aid will eventually have a child, either on their own or with medical assistance. Both men and women are equally likely to encounter fertility issues. In about one in every five infertile couples, both partners have contributing factors, and in approximately 15% of couples, no cause is discovered after all tests have been performed. This is known as **"unexplained infertility."** Infertility can be either primary or secondary.

Primary infertility occurs when someone is unable to conceive at all.

Secondary infertility occurs when a person has previously conceived but is no longer able to.

Infertility Reasons

Infertility is described as the inability to become pregnant after 12 months of trying. Any person of either sex who meets this description is infertile.

Causes Among Males

Male infertility can be caused by the following: **Problems with semen and sperm:** Semen is the milky fluid released by the penis after ejaculation, which contains both fluid and sperm. The fluid originates in the prostate gland, seminal vesicle, and other sex glands. Sperm is produced in the testicles. When the ejaculate exits the penis, semen helps transfer the sperm to the egg. A sperm count of less than 15 million, insufficient sperm motility, or sperm with a unique shape can all make it more difficult for sperm to fertilize the egg.

Approximately 2% of males may have sperm problems.

They may result from A medical condition: This could refer to a testicular infection, cancer, or surgery. Overheated testicles can be caused by an undescended testicle, a varicocele, a varicose vein in the scrotum, sauna or hot tub use, wearing tight clothing, or working in hot surroundings.

Ejaculation disorders: If the ejaculatory ducts become obstructed, semen may be ejaculated into the bladder. Hormonal imbalance: Hypogonadism, for example, can cause testosterone insufficiency.

Other Causes Could Include Genetic Factors: A male should have both X and Y chromosomes. If a person has two X chromosomes and one Y chromosome, as in Klinefelter syndrome, their testicles will grow improperly, resulting in insufficient testosterone, a low sperm count, or no sperm.

Mumps: If this develops after puberty, inflammation of the testicles might impair sperm production. **Hypospadias:** In this congenital defect, the urethral entrance is beneath the penis rather than at its tip.

Typically, doctors surgically repair this issue during infancy. If the repair is not completed, the sperm may have a more difficult time reaching the female's cervix. Hypospadias affects around one out of every 200 newborn males in the United States.

Cystic fibrosis is a chronic condition that causes the production of sticky mucus. This mucus primarily affects the lungs, but males may have a missing vas deferens. The vas deferens transports sperm from the epididymis to the ejaculatory duct and urethra.

Radiation therapy or chemotherapy. These medications can both reduce sperm production. Radiation therapy severity is typically determined by how close to the testicles the radiation was delivered.

Other Diseases: Anemia, Cushing's syndrome, diabetes, and thyroid disorders have all been associated with decreased fertility in males.

Drugs: Certain drugs raise the risk of male reproductive difficulties. These drugs include sulfasalazine (Azulfidine) and anabolic steroids.

Causes Among Females

Infertility in women can have a variety of causes. Problems with ovulation Ovulation problems account for around 25% of all infertility occurrences in females. Ovulation is the release of an egg once a month. The eggs may never be released, or they may be released just during specific cycles.

Ovulation Abnormalities Can Be Caused By: Hyperprolactinemia: If a woman's prolactin levels are high and she is not pregnant or lactating, it can interfere with ovulation and fertility.

Thyroid Problems: An overactive or underactive thyroid gland can cause a hormonal imbalance that prevents conception.

Polycystic ovarian syndrome (PCOS) is a hormonal disorder that can cause frequent or prolonged menstruation and interfere with ovulation.

Problems in the uterus or fallopian tubes can also hinder the egg from passing from the ovary to the uterus, or womb. If the egg does not migrate, it may be more difficult to conceive naturally.

Other Causes Other Factors Are:

Chronic conditions including AIDS and cancer.

Primary ovarian insufficiency (POI) occurs when the ovaries stop performing properly before the age of 40. Poor egg quality can impede conception. As a female ages, the amount and quality of her eggs drop.

Damaged eggs or those with genetic defects may be unable to support a pregnancy. The older a female is, the greater the risk. Pelvic surgery can occasionally result in scarring or damage to the fallopian tubes. Cervical surgery can sometimes result in scarring or shortening of the cervix. The cervix is the uterus' neck.

Submucosal fibroids are benign or noncancerous tumors that form in the uterine muscle wall. They can interfere with implantation or block. The fallopian tube blocks sperm from fertilizing the egg.

Endometriosis occurs when cells that ordinarily form within the uterine lining begin to proliferate elsewhere in the body.

Tubal ligation: In females who have elected to have their fallopian tubes shut, the procedure can be reversed, although the chances of becoming fertile again are slim.

Risk Factors

Certain risk factors enhance the likelihood of infertility in both sexes.

This Includes Smoking: Smoking increases considerably. It increases the risk of infertility in both sexes and may reduce the effectiveness of reproductive treatment. Smoking when pregnant increases the likelihood of pregnancy loss. Passive smoking has been linked to reduced fertility.

Chemotherapy: Certain chemotherapy medicines can cause ovarian failure or a severe reduction in sperm count. Radiation: If it is directed at the reproductive organs, it can raise the chance of fertility issues.

Sexually Transmitted Infections (STIs): Chlamydia can cause fallopian tube damage in women and scrotal inflammation in men. Other sexually transmitted infections may also cause infertility.

Age: The female's capacity to conceive may begin to decline progressively before or around the age of 35, whereas male fertility begins to decline after the age of 40.

In addition, other factors may be connected with infertility, albeit research in many cases is relatively limited.

This Includes Narcotics: Consuming drugs like cannabis or cocaine might reduce sperm count. Some females who use cannabis or cocaine may experience reproductive issues.

Chemical Exposure: Pesticides, herbicides, metals (such as lead), detergents, and solvents have all been related to fertility issues in both sexes. Obesity may diminish the chance of conceiving in both sexes.

Stress: Stress can play a role, especially if it causes decreased sexual activity. It can also influence female ovulation and male sperm production.

Exercise: Both men and women might experience reproductive issues as a result of excessive or insufficient exercise. It may affect male sperm count.

Nutrition: A bad diet can have an impact on fertility in both men and women. Fertility concerns may arise if an eating disorder causes severe weight loss.

Alcohol abuse: Excessive alcohol use might lower sperm count. It may also impair the efficacy of in vitro fertilization (IVF) therapies.

Infertility Therapy

Treatment to help a person conceive naturally will be determined by a variety of factors, including the person's age, length of infertility, personal preferences, and overall health.

The frequency of intercourse The first method that a couple seeking to conceive may want to try is to have sexual intercourse more frequently around the period of ovulation. Typically, the menstrual cycle lasts about 28-32 days. A female will typically ovulate between days 11 and 21 after the first day of her last cycle. Anyone with a cycle that lasts less than 21 days or more than 35 days should consult their doctor.

Other Treatments.

However, timing intercourse alone may not be enough to help a couple conceive.

Treatments will be based on the underlying reason for infertility. In guys, this may include erectile dysfunction drugs.

Surgery may include the removal of a varicose vein in the scrotum or the treatment of a clogged epididymis.

Females might be prescribed fertility medications to regulate or induce ovulation. These may include clomiphene (Clomid, Serophene), letrozole (Femara), dopamine agonists, and several hormonal medicines. If the fallopian tubes are obstructed or scarred, surgical treatment may allow eggs to travel through.

An individual may also be advised to undergo IVF. Doctors may also use laparoscopic surgery to treat endometriosis. They create a small incision in the abdomen and insert a thin, flexible microscope with a light at the end, known as a laparoscope. The surgeon can then remove the implants and scar tissue, perhaps reducing pain and improving fertility.

Assisted Conception

There are now the following procedures for assisted or artificial conception:

Intrauterine Insemination (IUI): At the time of ovulation, a doctor inserts a tiny catheter through the cervix into the uterus to collect a sperm sample directly.

In Vitro Fertilization: Doctors combine the sperm and unfertilized eggs in a petri dish, where fertilization can occur. They then implant the embryo in the uterus to start the pregnancy.

Intracytoplasmic sperm injection (ICSI) and assisted hatching are both examples of IVF methods.

Sperm Or Egg Donation: If necessary, a person can donate eggs or sperm. IVF can be used for fertility treatment involving donor eggs. Electric or vibratory stimulation can help a person achieve ejaculation. This can aid a male who is unable to ejaculate regularly, such as due to spinal cord damage.

Surgical sperm aspiration involves removing sperm from a component of the male reproductive tract such as the vas deferens, testicle, or epididymis. Doctors will utilize IVF to fertilize the egg or freeze the sperm for future use. Infertility diagnosis.

If a person has not conceived after 12 months of trying, he or she should consult a doctor. If the female partner is over 35 years old, the pair may want to consult a doctor sooner, as fertility tests can take time.

For example, a person over 35 may want to see a doctor after 6 months, whereas someone over 40 may want to see a doctor as soon as they notice they are not pregnant. A doctor can offer guidance and do preliminary assessments. The doctor may inquire about a person's sexual habits and provide advice accordingly. Tests are available, however they do not always identify a specific cause.

Male Infertility Tests

The doctor will ask about your medical history, medications, and sexual practices before doing a physical examination. If a test reveals an anomaly, the doctor may prescribe that the testicles be examined for lumps or abnormalities, as well as the shape and structure of the penis.

Additionally, The Doctor May Prescribe The Following Tests:

Semen Analysis: A sample can be collected to determine sperm concentration, motility, color, and quality, as well as the presence of blood or infection. Sperm counts change, thus many samples may be required. The lab will conduct a blood test to determine testosterone and other hormone levels.

Ultrasound: This can detect problems such as ejaculatory duct occlusion or retrograde ejaculation.

Chlamydia test: Although chlamydia can impair fertility, medications can treat it. However, antibiotics cannot reverse pre-existing reproductive harm.

Female Infertility Tests

A female will get a general physical examination in which the doctor will inquire about her medical history, medications, menstrual cycle, and sexual activities. They will also get a gynecologic exam and a variety of tests:

Blood tests can determine hormone levels and if a female is ovulating.

Hysterosalpingography: A technician injects fluid into the uterus and takes X-rays to see if the fluid flows appropriately out of the uterus and into the fallopian tubes. If a blockage exists, surgery may be required.

Laparoscopy: A thin, flexible tube with a camera at the end is introduced into the belly and pelvis, allowing the doctor to examine the fallopian tubes, uterus, and ovaries. This may indicate endometriosis, scarring, obstructions, and other uterine and fallopian tube anomalies.

Other testing may include ovarian reserve testing to count eggs after ovulation.

Pelvic ultrasonography is used to get a picture of the uterus and ovaries.

Thyroid function tests may alter hormonal balance. Couples with reproductive issues and those who want to have children later in life now have more options than ever before.

The first IVF-conceived child was born in 1978. Today, around 2.1% of all infants born in the United States each year are conceived with assisted reproductive technology (ART). Fertility treatment is becoming more accessible as new technology is developed, and success rates and safety are constantly improving.

CHAPTER 2

Diagnosis

Before infertility testing, your healthcare team or clinic will try to understand your sexual behaviors. They may give recommendations to boost your chances of becoming pregnant. However, in other infertile couples, no definite cause is identified. That is known as unexplained infertility. Infertility testing may require unpleasant treatments. It can also be pricey. Some medical insurance plans may not cover the cost of reproductive therapy.

Furthermore, there is no guarantee that you will become pregnant, even after all of the testing and counseling.

Tests for Male

Male fertility depends on the testicles producing enough healthy sperm. The sperm must be discharged from the penis into the vagina and transported to the egg.

Male infertility tests are designed to evaluate whether any of these processes have curable complications. A physical exam may include an inspection of your genitals. Specific infertility tests may include a Semen examination. Your healthcare provider may request one or more sperm samples. Masturbation or stopping sex to ejaculate into a clean container are frequent ways to collect sperm. A lab will then evaluate your sperm sample. In certain cases, urine may be tested to see if it contains sperm.

Hormonal testing. A blood test may be performed to evaluate the levels of testosterone and other male hormones. Genetics testing. This can be done to identify whether a genetic defect causes infertility. A testicular biopsy. This treatment involves removing a little sample of testicular tissue so that a lab can examine it under a microscope.

A biopsy is rarely required during infertility testing. It may be used in rare cases to determine whether there is a blockage in the reproductive system that prevents sperm from exiting the body in semen. This diagnosis is usually made based on your medical history, physical exam, and lab results.

A biopsy may also be performed to diagnose disorders that lead to infertility. Alternatively, it could be used to collect sperm for assisted reproductive techniques like in vitro fertilization. Imaging. In some situations, your healthcare provider may propose tests that produce images of the inside of your body. Ultrasound, for example, can detect issues in the scrotum, the glands that produce semen, or the tube that transports sperm from the testicles.

A brain MRI can detect benign pituitary gland cancers. These tumors can cause the gland to produce an excessive amount of the hormone prolactin, resulting in fewer or no sperm production.

Additional Testing. In rare situations, additional tests may be performed to assess the quality of your sperm. For example, a sperm sample may need to be tested for DNA abnormalities that could harm the sperm.

Tests For Women

Women's fertility depends on their ovaries delivering healthy eggs. The reproductive tract must allow an egg to move into the fallopian tubes and combine with sperm. The fertilized egg must then go to the uterus where it will connect to the lining.

Tests for female infertility attempt to identify issues with any of these phases. You may be subjected to a physical examination, which includes a routine pelvic examination. Infertility testing can include Ovulation tests. A blood test checks hormone levels to detect whether you ovulate. Thyroid function tests. If your doctor suspects that your infertility is caused by a thyroid condition, you can have this blood test.

If the gland produces too much or too little thyroid hormone, it may cause problems with fertility. Hysterosalpingography. Hysterosalpingography (his-tur-o-sal-ping-GOG-ruh-fee) examines the state of the uterus and fallopian tubes. It also checks for obstructions in the fallopian tubes and other issues. A special dye is injected into the uterus, and an X-ray is obtained.

Ovarian Reserve Testing. This allows your care team to determine how many eggs you have for ovulation. The procedure frequently begins with hormone testing early in the menstrual cycle. Other hormonal testing. These measure the levels of hormones that regulate ovulation. They also examine pituitary hormones, which regulate reproductive processes.

Imaging Testing. Pelvic ultrasonography detects disorders of the uterus or ovaries. A saline infusion ultrasonography is occasionally used to examine details inside the uterus that are not visible with conventional ultrasound. The saline infusion test is also known as a sonohysterogram (son-o-his-ter-OH-gram).

Occasionally, testing may include Hysteroscopy. Depending on your symptoms, your healthcare provider may do a hysteroscopy (his-ter-os-ko-pee) to look for a uterine condition. During the operation, a thin, illuminated probe is inserted through the cervix into the uterus to look for any abnormal indications. It can also be used to guide minor surgeries.

Laparoscopy. A tiny cut beneath the navel is used during laparoscopy. Thin viewing equipment is then inserted through the cut to examine the fallopian tubes, ovaries, and uterus. The treatment may reveal endometriosis, scarring, obstructions, or other problems with the fallopian tubes. It may also identify curable issues with the ovaries and uterus.

Laparoscopy is a surgical procedure that can also be used to address specific disorders. For example, it can be used to remove fibroids and endometriosis tissue. Not everyone requires all, or even several, of these tests before the cause of infertility is determined. You and your healthcare team pick which tests to have and when.

Infertility therapy depends on The cause of infertility. How long have you been infertile? If you have a partner, include their age as well as your own.

Personal Preferences. Some causes of infertility cannot be treated. If pregnancy does not occur after a year of unprotected sex, couples can typically conceive using infertility treatments known as assisted reproductive technology (ART). However, treatment might require significant financial, physical, emotional, and time obligations.

Treatment For Men

Men's treatment for general sexual issues or a lack of healthy sperm can include Lifestyle change.

Your healthcare provider may advise you to take the following steps.

Have intercourse more frequently and closer to ovulation.

Take frequent exercise.

Reduce your alcohol consumption or quit smoking.

Stop using fertility-affecting medications if your doctor tells you to.

Medicines. Your doctor may recommend medications to improve sperm count and increase the likelihood of a successful pregnancy. These prescription medicines may also help the testicles operate more effectively. Surgery. Sometimes surgery can cure a sperm barrier and restore fertility. In some situations, correcting a big varicocele may increase the overall chances of pregnancy.

Sperm retrieval methods. If you are unable to ejaculate or if there is no sperm in your semen, these approaches can be used to gather sperm. Sperm retrieval treatments may also be employed when assisted reproductive approaches are being considered when sperm levels are low or irregular.

Treatment For Women

Some women can enhance their fertility with just one or two treatments. Others may require multiple types of therapy to become pregnant. Fertility medications. These are the most common therapies for ovulation-related infertility. They can assist the ovaries release an egg if ovulation is inconsistent or ceases to occur.

Consult with your healthcare team about your choices. Inquire about the benefits and hazards of each form of fertility treatment.

Intrauterine Insemination, Or IUI. IUI involves inserting healthy sperm straight into the uterus around the time the ovary releases one or more eggs to be fertilized. Depending on the cause of infertility, IUI can be timed with your menstrual cycle or with the use of fertility medications. Your partner or a donor supplies the sperm.

Surgery To Restore Fertility. Hysteroscopy can cure certain uterine problems. These include polyps, scar tissue, and certain fibroids. Endometriosis, pelvic adhesions, and bigger fibroids may require either laparoscopic surgery with small cuts or standard surgery with a major cut in the stomach.

Assisted Reproductive Technology (ART) refers to any fertility procedure in which the egg and sperm are treated. The most often used ART treatment is in vitro fertilization (IVF).

Some of the major steps in an IVF cycle are: Fertility medications assist the ovaries produce eggs. Mature eggs are extracted from the ovaries. The eggs are fertilized with sperm in a laboratory dish. The fertilized eggs, also known as embryos, are implanted in the uterus. Embryos can also be preserved for later use.

In IVF cycles, other procedures may be used, including intracytoplasmic sperm injection (ICSI). A single, healthy sperm is inserted straight into a mature egg. ICSI is commonly performed when the quality or quantity of sperm is low. It may also be utilized if previous IVF rounds did not result in successful fertilization. Assisted hatching. This procedure facilitates an embryo's attachment to the uterine lining. It opens part of the embryo's outer coat, hence the name hatching. Donor egg or sperm.

ART is often performed utilizing a couple's eggs and sperm. You can, however, use donated eggs or sperm instead. This is an option if you are single or in a same-sex relationship. It is also done for medical purposes. These include age-related egg quality issues and sperm abnormalities such as an obstruction in the reproductive canal.

Donor eggs or sperm may also be used if one couple has a genetic illness that could be passed down to the baby. Donated embryos can also be used by infertile couples. These are from other couples that underwent infertility therapy and had leftover embryos frozen.

A gestational carrier. People who do not have a functioning uterus or for whom pregnancy poses a major health risk may choose IVF using a gestational carrier. In this situation, the couple's embryo is implanted in the uterus of a person willing to carry the pregnancy.

Genetic testing. Embryos created through IVF can be examined for genetic abnormalities. This is known as preimplantation genetic testing. Embryos that do not appear to have a genetic issue can be implanted in the uterus. This reduces the likelihood of a parent passing on a genetic problem to their child.

Treatment-related complications Complications of infertility therapy could include Multiple pregnancies. The most common side effect of infertility treatment is multiple pregnancies – twins, triplets, or more. A larger number of unborn infants in the womb increases the likelihood of early labor and delivery. It also increases the risk of pregnancy complications, such as gestational diabetes.

Babies who are born prematurely have a higher risk of health and developmental issues. Before beginning treatment, consult with your healthcare provider about all of the risks associated with multiple pregnancies. Ovarian hyperstimulation syndrome (OHSS).

Fertility medications can cause ovaries to become enlarged and painful. The risk of OHSS increases with the use of assisted reproductive technologies such as in vitro fertilization.

Symptoms may include mild stomach pain, bloating, and an upset stomach lasting approximately a week. If you get pregnant, your nausea may linger longer. Rarely, a more severe form of OHSS causes rapid weight gain and shortness of breath. This is an emergency that must be handled in a hospital. Bleeding or infection. Assisted reproductive technology or reproductive surgery carries the danger of bleeding or infection.

Coping And Supporting

Coping with infertility can be exceedingly challenging because there are so many unknowns. The path can be extremely emotionally draining.

Here Are Some Strategies To Help You Cope:

Be Prepared. The uncertainty surrounding infertility testing and treatment can be frustrating. Ask your fertility doctor to explain each step and how to prepare for them.

Set limits. Before you begin treatment, evaluate which procedures and how many you can financially and emotionally tolerate. Infertility treatments can be costly and are frequently not covered by insurance providers.

Furthermore, a successful pregnancy is frequently the result of multiple therapy attempts.

Consider Other Choices. You may need to employ donated sperm, eggs, or a gestational carrier. You could also consider adopting or not having children. Consider these choices as early as feasible in your infertility evaluation. It may reduce anxiety throughout therapy and feelings of despondency if you do not become pregnant.

Seek Help. Before, during, or after treatment, consider joining an infertile support group or consulting with a counselor. It can help you get through the procedure and cope with grief if your treatment fails.

Managing The Emotional Impact Of The Outcome Regardless of the outcome, you may face emotional issues. Not becoming pregnant or experiencing a miscarriage. Even in the most loving and supportive couples, the burden of not being able to have a kid can be unbearable.

Success. Even if fertility therapy is effective, it is normal to have worry and anxiety about failure during pregnancy. If you've already suffered from sadness or anxiety, you're more likely to experience them again in the months following your child's birth.

Multiple Births. A successful pregnancy with multiple births might cause stress both during and after delivery. Seek professional support from a therapist if the emotional burden of infertility treatment, pregnancy, or parenthood becomes too much for you or your partner.

Preparing For The Appointment

Depending on your age and health history, your primary care physician may prescribe a medical evaluation. A gynecologist, urologist, or family doctor can assist you in determining whether you need to see a specialist or a clinic that specializes in infertility treatments.

In some circumstances, you and your spouse may require a comprehensive infertility evaluation.

What You Can Do: To Prepare For Your First Appointment:

Take notes on your attempts to become pregnant.

Write down when you began trying to conceive and how frequently you've had sex, particularly around the midpoint of your menstrual cycle - the time of ovulation.

Bring your important medical information. Include any other medical concerns you or your partner have, as well as any previous infertility assessments or therapies.

Make a note of all the medications, vitamins, herbs, and any supplements you take.

Include the amounts you take (called dosages) and how frequently you take them. Make a list of questions to ask your healthcare providers. If time is limited, prioritize the most crucial queries.

For Infertility, Some Basic Questions To Ask Your Care Team Are:

What types of testing are required to determine why we have not conceived yet?

Which treatment would you recommend we try first?

What side effects could that treatment have?

What are the chances of having multiple babies with this treatment?

How many times should we try this procedure before conceiving?

If the first treatment fails, what would you propose attempting next?

Are there any long-term risks associated with this or other infertility treatments?

Feel free to ask your healthcare provider to repeat facts or ask follow-up questions.

What To Expect From Your Doctor:

Prepare to answer any questions your health care practitioner may ask. Your responses can help your doctor determine what tests and treatments you may require.

Questions For Couples

You and your partner may be asked some of the following questions:

How long have you been trying to become pregnant?

How frequently do you have sex?

Do you use lubricants during sex?

Do either of you smoke?

Do either of you consume alcohol or recreational drugs? How often?

Do either of you take any medications, nutritional supplements, or anabolic steroids?

Have either of you had treatment for any other medical conditions, including sexually transmitted infections?

Questions For Men

Your health care expert might ask:

Do you struggle to gain muscle mass, or do you use any supplements to help you do so?

Do you ever sense fullness in your scrotum, particularly after standing for a long time?

Do you have any testicular pain or soreness after ejaculation?

Have you ever struggled to maintain an erection, ejaculated too quickly, were unable to ejaculate, or experienced reduced sexual desire?

Have you ever had a child with any previous partners? Do you regularly take hot or steam baths?

Questions For The Woman

Your healthcare expert might ask:

What age did you first experience menstruation?

What do your regular cycles look like?

How regular, lengthy, and hefty are they?

Have you ever become pregnant before?

Have you been tracking your periods or checking for ovulation? If so, how many cycles?

What's your regular daily diet? Do you get any exercise? How often?

CHAPTER 3

Dealing With Mental Stress During Treatment

Dealing with mental stress, particularly in the context of reproductive issues, is critical for general well-being and can benefit the fertility journey.

Here's A Complete Approach To Efficiently Managing And Mitigating Mental Stress.

1. Acknowledge your emotions. Validate feelings: Recognize that feelings of grief, frustration, anger, and anxiety are common reactions to fertility issues. It is critical to recognize these emotions rather than suppress them. Accepting the journey: Recognize that the fertility process can be unpredictable and emotionally draining. Accepting this can help you deal with the stress.

2. Seek Professional Help. Therapists and counselors: Consult a therapist or counselor who specializes in infertility and reproductive health. They can help you manage stress, cope with emotions, and provide support. Support groups: Join infertility support groups to discuss

your stories and get emotional support from people who understand what you're going through.

3. Open communication with your partner. Share your feelings: Regularly discuss your feelings and worries with your partner. Maintaining an open discussion ensures that both partners understand and can support one another. Joint Decisions: Make fertility decisions together. This shared responsibility can lessen individual stress and promote teamwork.

4. Practice relaxation techniques. Mindfulness and Meditation: Practices such as mindfulness meditation can help to reduce anxiety and promote emotional health. Apps such as Headspace and Calm provide guided sessions for stress alleviation.

Deep breathing exercises: Simple practices, such as deep breathing, can instantly reduce stress and promote relaxation. Yoga: Including yoga in your regimen can benefit your physical and mental wellness. Fertility yoga focuses primarily on relaxation and reproductive health.

5. Maintain a healthy lifestyle. Balanced Diet: Consuming a good diet helps boost mood and energy levels. Include a variety of fruits, veggies, lean proteins, and nutritious grains. Regular exercise produces endorphins, which are natural mood enhancers. Aim for

regular, moderate activity, such as walking, swimming, or biking. Adequate Sleep: Make sure you get enough restful sleep every night, as inadequate sleep can worsen stress and harm your health.

6. Set realistic expectations. Manage expectations: Recognize that fertility treatments can be a lengthy and uncertain procedure. Setting reasonable expectations might assist in alleviating disappointment and stress. Focus on Small Wins: Celebrate little milestones and development rather than focusing solely on the overall objective.

7. Limit Stressful Triggers. Avoid overexposure to social media. Limit your time spent on social media, which can sometimes elicit unpleasant emotions, particularly when viewing pregnancy announcements or infant images. Set boundaries: Politely decline to attend emotionally stressful occasions, such as baby showers or family reunions where you may be asked about having children.

8. Engage in enjoyable activities. Hobbies and Interests: Engage in hobbies and activities that you enjoy that will help you forget about fertility troubles. This could be reading, drawing, gardening, or cooking. Socialize: Spend time with friends and family who offer good encouragement and friendship.

9. Educational Resources. Inform yourself: Uncertainty-induced anxiety can be reduced by learning more about infertility and its treatment.

Read books, watch webinars, and consult credible sources. Avoid information overload: While remaining informed is crucial, don't overload yourself with information. Balance your research with leisure.

10. Practice self-compassion. Be Kind to Yourself: Treat yourself with the same compassion and understanding that you would show a friend in a similar position. Recognize your accomplishments and strengths. Forgive yourself: Recognize that having terrible days and setbacks is normal.

Forgive yourself for any perceived failures and keep going forward.

11. Spiritual and Religious Support. Faith-Based Support: If you are religious or spiritual, doing prayer, meditation, or other spiritual practices might help you relax and reduce stress. Many faith communities provide support groups and counseling services to couples experiencing infertility.

12. Professional Stress Management Techniques. Cognitive Behavioral Therapy (CBT) can help you

change negative thought patterns and enhance your emotional responses to stress.

Biofeedback: This approach allows you to gain awareness and control over physiological functions such as heart rate and muscle tension to relieve stress. Managing mental stress during reproductive issues is critical for both emotional well-being and the effectiveness of fertility treatments.

Recognizing your emotions, seeking professional help, keeping open communication with your partner, practicing relaxation techniques, and engaging in healthy lifestyle choices will help you manage stress and navigate the reproductive path more effectively

These and other healthy practices can boost your mood and help you focus on living your life.

CHAPTER 4

Lifestyle Modifications To Improve Fertility

Keys to Fertility The keys to fertility for both men and women include keeping a healthy weight, exercising, and eating foods that help you conceive and get pregnant. Extreme weight has been linked to 30% of infertility cases. Obese women are three times more likely to become infertile.

Women who are overweight can increase their fertility by decreasing only 5% of their body weight. Insulin resistance leads the body to secrete more insulin, which prevents ovulation.

Ovulation issues are common in underweight women. Obesity in men changes testosterone and other hormones, which can impact sperm count and mobility. Sperm-related infertility is responsible for up to 33% of male factor infertility.

In addition to diet, lifestyle behaviors that encourage conceptions include minimizing alcohol intake, eliminating smoking, and engaging in moderate daily exercise. Healthy eating can improve fertility. What you consume has an impact on the health of your or your partner's eggs and sperm.

Proper dietary adjustments can reduce women's risk of infertility caused by ovulation issues by 80%

Consuming full-fat dairy lowers the risk of ovarian dysfunction and promotes healthy ovulation.

Avoid low-fat dairy products because studies have shown that they induce ovulatory disruption.

Consume protein from meat and vegetables.

Avoid consuming too much animal protein, as it raises the chance of infertility.

Consuming soy can improve female fertility.

Men should avoid soy since it can diminish sperm counts.

Eat extra fiber.

Eat dark leafy greens to promote ovulation and produce healthy sperm.

Include beans in your diet since they promote fertility.

Including walnuts in your man's diet can increase his fertility.

Avoid trans fats, which are linked to a higher risk of infertility.

Avoid eating highly processed meals and hydrogenated oils.

Reduce your intake of carbohydrates and sweets.

Consume complex carbohydrates to help regulate blood sugar levels. High blood sugar levels have been linked to reduced conception.

Moderate caffeine consumption, about 1-2 cups per day, has little effect on fertility. Higher dosages may. The science isn't conclusive.

Prenatal Vitamins Take a multivitamin or prenatal vitamin designed to give the nutrients required for proper hormone function, egg formation, and fetal growth.

Prenatal vitamins include folate, vitamins A and D, iron, B6, and B12. These nutrients are the foundation of a healthy pregnancy.

Folate from diet alone is insufficient. Folate from nutritional supplements can improve pregnancy outcomes.

Women should take 800 mcg of folate per day during fertility treatments and pregnancy.

Take iron supplements. According to studies, women who took iron supplements daily were 40% less likely to have trouble conceiving. Sperm retained in the body is susceptible to oxidative stress, which can damage sperm DNA.

Smoking, obesity, chronic disease, and reaching the age of 38 all increase the chance of sperm destruction. Antioxidants such as vitamin C, E, Folic Acid, Selenium, and Zinc can help prevent sperm destruction. Vitamin D is required for the production of sex hormones as well as ovarian function.

Lower vitamin D levels reduce sperm motility and, in women, are linked to pregnancy difficulties. A Yale study found that vitamin D insufficiency is connected to infertility.

Improving Vitamin D levels has been demonstrated to increase IVF success rates.

Vitamin E is related to better reproductive results. It can reduce the time to pregnancy and enhance sperm motility. However, use these supplements with caution because large dosages can be harmful. Omega-3 fatty acids assist control of hormones, increase ovulation, and improve blood flow to the reproductive organs.

Exercise Moderate exercise (up to an hour) can lower the risk of infertility and increase sperm quality. Poor sperm quality might lead to miscarriages. Exercise lasting fewer than 15 minutes may raise the chance of infertility. Extreme activity can result in infertility. Your fitness habits can also have an impact on your IVF outcome.

Dental Health Oral health is important. Gum disease, cavities, and periodontitis have a deleterious impact on pregnancy. Quit smoking. According to studies, smoking raises the risk of infertility by 13%.

Smoking can increase the time it takes to conceive. Smoking raises the risk of miscarriage and can cause birth abnormalities. Alcohol can have an impact on both male and female fertility, including conception and implantation. There is no safe amount of alcohol.

Stress Stress reduces fertility.

Acupuncture, yoga, meditation, deep breathing, and other mind-body therapies may be beneficial. Massage can also assist.

Timing Intercourse. Understanding your reproductive cycle might increase your chances of conceiving. Although timing intercourse can help in conception, it does not affect fertility.

Lubricants It is well known that some water-based lubricants, as well as any lubricant containing spermicide, should be avoided. There are sperm-friendly lubricants that will not impair sperm motility.

Sleep Melatonin is naturally created by the body when asleep. Any artificial light, including gadget screen light, might influence melatonin production. Sleep lowers cortisol levels, which can reduce testosterone.

Men can boost their fertility by avoiding tight-fitting garments, long bike rides, and hot tubs, as well as keeping a laptop in their lap, which can raise scrotal temperature and lower sperm production.

CHAPTER 5

The Fertility Journey: Emotional Wellbeing And Resilience

A reproductive journey is undeniably emotional, and it is critical to emphasize mental wellness and resilience. It is important to remember that the reproductive journey is unique to each individual. By combining several ways, you will be able to efficiently manage your emotional well-being, build resilience, and handle the complexities of the journey with a more capable and balanced mentality.

Understanding Emotional Impact

Understanding how fertility issues affect emotions is critical for maintaining emotional health. When dealing with the complexities of the fertility road, people experience a variety of emotions, including despair, stress, guilt, and solitude.

Recognizing these feelings and understanding that they are natural in the given circumstances is critical.

Validation Of Emotion: Understand that experiencing various emotions during fertility trials is normal. Validating your feelings allows you to manage them without criticism and fosters self-compassion.

Normalizing Responses: Recognize that many people with fertility troubles are depressed, stressed, or guilty. Normalizing these behaviors can help people feel less isolated and more connected.

Seeking Support: Discuss your problems with your partner, friends, or relatives. The need for assistance provides a means of self-expression and reinforces that you do not have to face life alone.

Professional Guidance: It is recommended that you contact a mental health practitioner who specializes in fertility-related emotional disorders. They can provide coping skills, perspective, and a vibrant environment.

Patience With Yourself: Be kind and gentle to yourself. The fertility route is complicated, and emotions take time to process. Allow yourself adequate space to process these emotions without setting an unattainable ideal.

Communication With Spouse: Maintain close communication with your spouse. Emotional disclosure strengthens the emotional bond, encouraging reciprocity of emotional support and understanding.

Setting Boundaries: Set boundaries for conversations about fertility. This allows you to choose the story and how you handle the emotional parts of the trip.

Engaging In Self-care: Choose self-care activities that promote comfort and relaxation. Practicing mindfulness, meditation, or leisure activities improves emotional well-being. Individuals and couples who recognize and understand the emotional element of fertility difficulties can take control of their well-being, develop a support network, and manage the fertility route with resilience and kindness to themselves.

Building Resilience For The Fertility Journey
Developing resilience is critical for dealing with the emotional complexities of the fertility journey. Resilience is the ability to adapt successfully to adversity, and it is essential for maintaining emotional well-being during the stages of conception.

Resilience development is an ongoing process that includes accepting emotional challenges, seeking help, and developing appropriate coping mechanisms. Individuals and couples who demonstrate resilience can weather the reproductive journey with greater emotional strength, adaptability, and a sense of control. Here's how. Self-care is a need. Self-care is a vital part of dealing with emotional wellness, particularly during the reproductive process.

Here's How Different Self-care Habits Improve Physical And Mental Health:

1. Regular exercise promotes physical health by improving cardiovascular fitness, weight management, and muscle tone. Endorphins are neurotransmitters that are released during physical activity and work as natural mood enhancers, helping to manage stress, anxiety, and depression.

2. Balanced Diet: Physical Benefits: A balanced diet contains all important nutrients for optimal health, including reproductive health. Emotional Benefits: Nutrient-rich diets have a favorable influence on mood and energy levels, resulting in a stable emotional state.

3. Adequate Sleep: Quality sleep promotes physical healing and immune system function. Emotional Benefits: A lack of sleep may lead to increased stress and emotional volatility. Adequate rest is necessary for emotional health.

4. Relaxation Techniques (Yoga, Meditation): Physical Benefits: Yoga improves flexibility, balance, and overall wellness. Emotional Benefits: Meditation and yoga help to relax, reduce tension, and cultivate mindfulness, which leads to better emotional states.

5. Physical Benefits: Stress management reduces the impact of stress hormones on the body and promotes general wellness. Emotional Benefits: Stress management techniques like deep breathing and progressive muscle relaxation improve emotional resilience and stability.

Professional Support Professional counseling or treatment regulates the emotional component of reproductive difficulties.

Here's How Mental Health Specialists May Help During This Difficult Time:

1. Emotional Processing: Safe Space: Therapy provides a quiet space for individuals or couples to express their feelings about reproductive therapy. Validation: Mental health experts validate and normalize the full range of emotions, making people feel understood and accepted.

2. Coping strategies include tailored techniques. Therapists also offer coping skills specific to each

individual's requirements for dealing with fertility-related stress, worry, and emotional weight. Counseling helps people improve their emotional control skills, making the fertility process easier to handle.

3. Strengthening Relationships: Therapy can enhance communication and emotional support between couples. It helps us to face the issues together.

4. Exploration of Concerns: Identifying Underlying Issues: Mental health practitioners provide a safe space for individuals to address emotional concerns that may cause stress or impact fertility.

5. Counseling supports informed decision-making by addressing the emotional impact of reproductive treatment options for individuals or couples. Navigating Uncertainty: Therapists handle the uncertainty of the reproductive journey, allowing patients to make decisions that are appropriate for their emotional state.

Positive Mindset And Hope

A good perspective and hope are powerful forces that can significantly impact your reproductive journey.

Here's How

1. Empowerment and Sense of Control: A positive attitude empowers you by focusing on things you can control. It shifts the emphasis from impediments to active involvement in the march.

2. Celebrating Small wins: Recognizing Progress: Small wins, whether personal or positive in the reproductive journey, provide a sense of progress and accomplishment.

3. Gratitude Practices: Positive Reflection: Giving thanks involves reflecting on the positive aspects of your life and building a happy mindset. This approach can help to alleviate the challenges of the fertility journey.

4. Enhancing Resilience and Adaptability: A cheerful mindset promotes resilience. It encourages flexibility in the face of failure, resulting in better trip navigation with a more resilient and hopeful outlook.

5. Hope is a motivator that encourages action. Being able to embrace hope puts you on track to taking the proper

activities and trying out various reproductive treatments. It inspires perseverance and determination.

Looking For Support

However, receiving support is a vital and enabling step in the reproductive process.

Here's Why

1. Validation and Understanding: Sharing your emotions with loved ones or professionals provides emotional support. It helps you feel understood and less alone in your path.

2. Strengthening Relationships: Connecting with loved ones. Friendship, family, or partner support strengthens emotional bonds. It promotes sentiments of togetherness and similarity in relationships.

3. Reducing Isolation: Participating in support groups and online communities can help you connect with others facing similar issues. Sharing this experience reduces depersonalization and fosters a sense of connection.

4. Perspective and Guidance: Consulting mental health specialists provides professional guidance. Therapists or counselors can provide insightful comments, coping

strategies, and tailored recommendations to meet your specific requirements.

5. Share the Burden for Emotional Relief: Sharing your emotions with others helps to alleviate the emotional weight. Sharing both the highs and the lows results in a more balanced emotional environment.

CHAPTER 6

Fertility Challenges

Fertility problems are difficulties that a couple may encounter in establishing pregnancy or carrying a pregnancy to term. These difficulties might result from a multitude of causes impacting one or both couples.

Here's A Thorough Overview Of Frequent Reproductive Issues:

1. Ovulatory disorders. Polycystic Ovary Syndrome (PCOS) is a hormonal disease that causes irregular or no ovulation. The symptoms include irregular periods, increased hair growth, and acne.

Hypothalamic Dysfunction: Stress, considerable weight loss or gain, and extreme exercise can all disrupt hormone production and impact ovulation.

Premature Ovarian Insufficiency (POI): A loss in ovarian function before the age of 40, resulting in decreased egg production. Hyperprolactinemia is the overproduction of prolactin, which can impair ovulation.

2. Tubular Factors Blocked or damaged fallopian tubes may be caused by pelvic inflammatory disease (PID),

endometriosis, or prior procedures. Blocked tubes hinder sperm from reaching the egg and fertilized eggs from reaching the uterus.

Ectopic Pregnancy: A pregnancy that occurs outside of the uterus, generally in a fallopian tube, which can harm the tube and impair future fertility.

3. Cervical or Uterine Factors Uterine fibroids are non-cancerous growths in the uterus that can prevent fertilized egg implantation or cause miscarriages. Polyps are benign growths on the uterine lining that might disrupt implantation.

Congenital Anomalies: Abnormalities in the structure of the uterus, such as a septate uterus, might result in repeated miscarriages. Cervical Insufficiency: The cervix opens prematurely during pregnancy, resulting in miscarriage or preterm birth.

4. Endometriosis is a disorder in which tissue identical to the uterine lining grows outside it, typically on the ovaries, fallopian tubes, and other pelvic organs. This can lead to inflammation, scar tissue, and adhesions, all of which have an impact on fertility.

5. Male Factor Infertility. Low Sperm Count (Oligospermia): Less than 15 million sperm per milliliter

of semen. Poor Sperm Motility (Asthenozoospermia): Sperm that cannot swim far enough to reach the egg.

Aberrant Sperm Morphology (Teratozoospermia): Sperm that are aberrant in shape and may be unable to fertilize the egg. Varicocele: Enlarged veins in the scrotum that can heat the testicles and impair sperm production and quality.

Ejaculation Disorders: Examples include retrograde ejaculation, in which semen enters the bladder rather than escaping through the penis.

6. Unexplained infertility When no identifiable cause is found despite extensive testing of both couples. This can be frustrating, and it may necessitate multiple treatments to achieve pregnancy.

7. Age-related infertility.

Female Age: As women age, particularly after 35, the quantity and quality of their eggs diminish, making it more difficult to conceive and increasing the risk of miscarriage.

Male Age: While men generate sperm throughout their lives, sperm quality can deteriorate with age, reducing fertility and raising the chance of genetic defects.

8. Lifestyle Factors. Smoking impairs egg and sperm quality and raises the risk of miscarriage. Alcohol: Excessive alcohol intake can impair fertility in both men and women. Weight: Being overweight or underweight can have an impact on hormone production and ovulation. Stress: Can disrupt the hormonal signals that control ovulation and sperm production.

9. Environmental Factors. Toxic exposure: Pesticides, heavy metals, and other environmental contaminants can all have an impact on reproductive health. Cancer treatments, including radiation and chemotherapy, can decrease fertility in both men and women.

10. Genetic Factors. Genetic abnormalities like Klinefelter syndrome in men and Turner syndrome in women can impair reproductive ability.

Practical Suggestions On What Step To Take Next

Navigating fertility problems can be daunting, but with practical efforts and the correct support, couples can increase their chances of becoming pregnant.

Here Is A Thorough Guide On What To Do Next:

1. Understand Your Fertility Status. Track Ovulation: Use ovulation predictor kits (OPKs), basal body temperature charts, or fertility apps to determine when

you are most fertile. Monitor your menstrual cycle to spot any irregularities.

2. Consult a Healthcare Professional for Initial Assessment: For a preliminary evaluation, see your primary care physician or an obstetrician. If initial efforts fail, consult a reproductive endocrinologist (RE), who specializes in diagnosing and treating infertility.

3. Comprehensive Testing for Women: Blood tests: To determine hormone levels (FSH, LH, estrogen, progesterone, prolactin, thyroid hormones).

Ultrasound: Used to examine the ovaries and uterus for structural problems. Hysterosalpingography (HSG): An X-ray that looks for obstructions in the fallopian tubes.

Ovarian Reserve Testing: Estimates the amount and quality of leftover eggs. Laparoscopy is a minimally invasive procedure for detecting endometriosis or other pelvic diseases.

For Men: Semen analysis evaluates sperm count, motility, and morphology.

Hormone Testing: Checks testosterone and other hormone levels. hereditary Testing: If there are signs of hereditary problems with sperm production.

4. Lifestyle Modifications Healthy Diet: Consume a well-balanced diet rich in fruits, vegetables, lean proteins, and whole grains. Consider including fertility-boosting foods such as leafy greens, almonds, and seeds. Maintain a healthy weight. Both underweight and overweight conditions can have an impact on fertility. Aim for a BMI that falls within the normal range.

Exercise Moderately: While regular physical activity is healthy, avoid excessive or high-intensity exercise, as it can interrupt ovulation. To promote reproductive health, both spouses should quit smoking and restrict their alcohol intake. Reduce Stress: Engage in stress-reduction exercises such as yoga, meditation, or mindfulness.

5. Consider Fertility Treatments. Medications: Clomiphene Citrate (Clomid): Promotes ovulation in women with ovulatory problems. Gonadotropins are injectable hormones that stimulate ovulation. Metformin is used to treat PCOS by improving insulin resistance and ovulation. Intrauterine Insemination (IUI): Sperm is inserted directly into the uterus around the time of ovulation to facilitate conception. In Vitro Fertilization (IVF) is the process of retrieving eggs, fertilizing them in a lab, and transferring the resulting embryos to the uterus. Intracytoplasmic Sperm Injection (ICSI): During IVF, a single sperm is injected directly into an egg,

which is effective in treating severe male infertility. 6. Assess Financial and Emotional Support. Insurance Coverage: Check your health insurance policy to see if it covers reproductive treatments or drugs. Financial Planning: Speak with a financial advisor or the fertility clinic's financial counselor about payment plans, loans, or grants. Emotional Support: Seek counseling or participate in support groups to cope with the emotional hardship of infertility. Many clinics provide counseling services, and you can join local or online support groups.

7. Stay informed and advocate for yourself. Educate yourself. Read books, attend seminars, and participate in online forums to remain up to date on the newest fertility research and therapies. Ask questions: Don't be afraid to ask your healthcare professional about all feasible options and the reasoning for their advice. Second Opinions: If you're not sure about a diagnosis or treatment plan, get a second opinion from another professional.

8. Consider Alternative and Complementary Therapies. Acupuncture: Some studies suggest that acupuncture can boost fertility by increasing blood flow to the reproductive organs and harmonizing hormones. Herbal Supplements: Before taking any supplements, consult with a doctor to ensure they are safe and appropriate for your needs. Mind-Body Programs: Programs that include

relaxation techniques, stress management, and lifestyle counseling can improve general health and perhaps increase fertility.

9. Think about donor options and surrogacy. Donor Sperm or Eggs: If sperm or egg quality is a major concern, donor sperm or eggs may be a possibility. Surrogacy: When a woman is unable to carry a pregnancy, gestational surrogacy involves another woman carrying the pregnancy utilizing embryos from the intended parents or donors.

10. Adoption. Consider Adoption: If fertility treatments are unsuccessful or undesirable, adoption may be a rewarding road to motherhood. Couples who follow these steps and remain proactive have a better chance of overcoming reproductive issues and realizing their desire for children.

CHAPTER 7

Alternative And Complementary Treatments For Fertility Enhancement

Many people dream of bringing new life into the world. But for other couples, the path to parenthood can be difficult. To achieve this treasured goal, couples are increasingly resorting to alternative and complementary therapies for fertility enhancement.

These holistic treatments provide a natural and integrated approach to addressing fertility concerns and improving reproductive health. We'll look at a variety of alternative and complementary therapies that may improve fertility and general health.

Herbal Treatments For Fertility Enhancement

Herbal medicines have been utilized for millennia to promote reproductive health and alleviate fertility issues. Indeed, numerous "natural fertility boosters" have stood the test of time. However, many herbs have yet to be tested in verified clinical trials. That is why it is critical to consult a skilled herbalist and your healthcare provider before introducing herbs into your regimen, as their effects might vary and any interactions with drugs must be explored.

The Power Of Acupuncture

Acupuncture, an ancient Chinese treatment, is becoming popular as an alternative therapy for fertility improvement. This technique includes inserting small needles into certain spots on the body to regulate energy flow, or "qi." The theory is that acupuncture can improve reproductive health by restoring equilibrium to the body's energy channels.

According to studies, acupuncture may improve blood flow to the reproductive organs, reduce stress, and increase the likelihood of successful conception. While research is ongoing, many couples benefit from acupuncture's soothing and balancing benefits.

Acupuncture's potential benefits for fertility enhancement go beyond physiological consequences. Aside from the physical components, acupuncture provides a comprehensive approach that includes mental well-being.

Acupuncture sessions can promote relaxation and stress reduction, which can improve hormone balance and general reproductive health. Acupuncture promotes a sense of serenity and emotional harmony, creating an atmosphere conducive to conception. It's worth mentioning that, while individual experiences differ, acupuncture has gained popularity as a supplemental therapy to traditional reproductive therapies.

As couples travel the often difficult path to parenting, acupuncture can be a helpful tool due to its possible physiological effects and contribution to mental resilience during the fertility journey.

Yoga And Meditation For Fertility

Stress has a substantial impact on fertility because it disrupts hormonal balance and affects ovulation. Recognizing this, couples are turning to mind-body therapies like yoga and meditation to improve conception.

Yoga, a centuries-old practice, includes poses that increase flexibility and strength while also improving blood circulation to the pelvic area. Meditation, on the other hand, is an effective strategy for relaxing the mind, reducing anxiety, and improving emotional well-being.

Couples who incorporate these techniques into their routine can create a conducive atmosphere for conception while also supporting their emotional and physical well-being.

The Role Of Diet In Enhancement

What we consume influences our entire health, including reproductive health. A nutritious, well-balanced diet helps improve hormonal balance and fertility. Nutritional decisions can have an impact on menstrual regularity, egg and sperm health, and the overall environment for conception. Leafy greens, healthy grains, and antioxidant-rich meals are commonly suggested for their ability to improve egg quality and sperm health.

In contrast, limiting your intake of processed foods, coffee, and alcohol can improve your fertility. It is suggested that you consult a dietitian for individualized advice based on your fertility goals.

Chiropractic Care And Fertility

Chiropractic therapy, which is normally connected with musculoskeletal health, has recently acquired popularity as an alternate approach to fertility improvement. This therapy focuses on spine alignment and nervous system function, which may have an impact on reproductive health. Misalignments in the spine can alter nerve signals that govern reproductive organs, thereby impairing fertility. Chiropractic treatments try to restore appropriate nerve system function, which may benefit reproductive health. While further research is needed, several people have experienced favorable results when combining chiropractic care with traditional fertility therapies.

The Effects Of Drug Use On Reproductive Health

Drug use, whether recreational or prescribed, can have a substantial influence on your reproductive health and interrupt your path to parenting. The consequences of drug usage on fertility are seen in both illicit drugs and certain pharmaceuticals. They have the potential to alter hormonal balance, prevent ovulation and sperm production, and impair overall reproductive function.

Alcohol, smoking, and recreational drugs can all reduce fertility by altering hormone levels and lowering the quality of eggs and sperm. Certain prescription drugs used to treat chronic diseases may inadvertently disrupt fertility by producing hormonal imbalances or impairing reproductive organ function.

It is critical to understand that the decisions you make about drug usage might have long-term effects on your ability to conceive and carry a healthy pregnancy. If you want to improve your fertility, you should talk to a doctor about the potential risks of drug use and look into other methods that will help your reproductive health.

Embracing Holistic Pathways To Parenthood

Starting the journey to parenting with alternative and complementary therapies for conception enhancement can be a wonderful and empowering experience. Individuals and couples can improve their reproductive health and boost their chances of natural conception by nurturing their bodies, minds, and spirits. However, it is critical to pursue these therapies with realistic expectations and in conjunction with medical counsel, particularly for people with pre-existing diseases.

Incorporating herbal treatments, acupuncture, yoga, meditation, nutrition, and chiropractic therapy into one's regimen can result in a more comprehensive approach to fertility improvement. These therapies provide not only physical advantages but also promote mental well-being and develop the mind-body connection.

Remember that everyone's experience is unique, so what works for one person may not work for another. Maintaining open communication with healthcare doctors and holistic practitioners is critical for developing a thorough plan that is personalized to each individual's needs. The field of alternative and complementary therapies for fertility enhancement is vast and exciting.

These therapies, which range from ancient techniques like acupuncture to more modern approaches like chiropractic therapy, provide a variety of options for those looking for natural ways to improve reproductive health. Individuals and couples who embrace these comprehensive routes to motherhood can face infertility issues with hope and resilience.

CHAPTER 8

Importance Of Staying Proactive And Informed

Couples dealing with fertility issues must stay proactive and knowledgeable. This method entails actively managing and addressing fertility concerns, staying current on the newest research, and advocating for one's health.

Here's A Comprehensive Explanation Of The Significance Of Being Proactive And Informed:

1. Early Diagnosis and Intervention Early detection of reproductive difficulties allows for faster intervention, which can considerably increase the odds of successful therapy.

Better results: Addressing concerns like hormonal imbalances or structural difficulties as soon as possible will help to avoid complications and enhance overall reproductive health.

2. Improved Treatment Options. Make Informed Decisions: Being knowledgeable about various reproductive treatments allows couples to make informed selections based on their personal and medical situations. Tailored Treatments: Understanding various treatment protocols (e.g., IUI, IVF, ICSI) enables couples to debate and select the best options with their healthcare professional.

3. Optimized Health and Lifestyle Options Healthy Habits: Understanding the effects of nutrition, exercise, and lifestyle on fertility supports healthier choices, such as keeping a healthy weight, quitting smoking, and limiting alcohol intake.

Risk Reduction: By being aware of environmental toxins and other variables that can affect fertility, couples can reduce their exposure and limit risks.

4. Empowerment and Management Active Participation: Being proactive entails actively participating in one's fertility journey, from scheduling regular medical check-ups to asking crucial questions in consultations.

Sense of Control: Taking responsibility for fertility health can alleviate emotions of helplessness and increase a sense of control over the situation, which is beneficial to mental health.

5. Effective Communication with Health Care Providers Informed Conversations: Well-informed individuals can have more productive discussions with their doctors, ensuring that they understand their illness and the reasons for prescribed therapies. Advocacy: Knowledge enables couples to advocate for themselves, seeking second opinions as needed and ensuring their issues are handled.

6. Financial planning and management. Cost Awareness: Understanding the costs of various reproductive treatments and available financing solutions aids in better budgeting and spending management. Insurance Navigation: Understanding what insurance covers can help couples optimize their benefits and explore additional financial aid options if necessary.

7. Coping Strategies for Emotional and Psychological Support. Couples who are aware of the emotional impact of infertility and the availability of support tools such as counseling and support groups are better able to manage stress and emotional strain.

Community Support: Joining support groups and online communities offers emotional support, shared experiences, and practical help.

8. Keeping up with advancements. Keeping up with the latest reproductive research and technological breakthroughs can lead to new treatment options that were not previously available. Innovative Treatments: Learning about novel treatments, like genetic screening procedures or enhanced IVF protocols, can help increase success rates.

9. Long-term Health Considerations Preventive Care: By proactively managing fertility health, you can discover and manage other underlying health issues, such as hormone imbalances or chronic diseases, which improve overall health. Future Planning: Staying aware allows you to plan for future family-building possibilities, such as egg-freezing or exploring alternate paths to parenthood.

10. Informed risk assessment Understanding dangers: Knowing the potential dangers and side effects of various reproductive treatments enables couples to make informed decisions.

Balanced Expectations: Understanding success rates and potential hurdles assists in creating reasonable expectations and preparing for various outcomes.

Practical Steps To Stay Proactive And Informed

Educate Yourself: Read credible books, research articles, and internet resources about fertility and reproductive health.

Attend Seminars And Workshops: Attend fertility seminars, webinars, and workshops to learn from specialists and connect with other couples dealing with similar issues.

Join Support Groups. Connect with local or online support groups to share your experiences, and receive emotional support, and practical guidance.

Regular Medical Check-ups: Schedule and attend regular check-ups with your healthcare practitioner to monitor your reproductive health and handle any difficulties that arise.

Ask Questions: During medical appointments, ask questions to better understand your health, treatment options, and the reasoning behind medical advice.

Seek Second Opinions: If you are unsure about a diagnosis or treatment plan, don't hesitate to seek second opinions.

Stay Up To Date: Follow fertility clinics, research institutions, and professional associations to stay up to date on the newest reproductive treatments and research.

Track Your Health: Use fertility apps or notebooks to keep track of your menstrual cycles, ovulation, and any symptoms so you can submit precise information to your doctor.

Couples who are proactive and aware can better navigate the complicated landscape of fertility issues, increasing their chances of a successful pregnancy and preserving overall well-being.

CHAPTER 9

Supporting Your Partner On A Fertility Journey

Fertility journeys may be extremely tiring, both physically and emotionally, and knowing how to assist your spouse can help them cope. I want to make sure you and your spouse have the tools you need to talk about your fertility and plans; I've highlighted various ways you can support one another emotionally and logistically below.

Emotional Support: Listen Your companion may need to discuss their experience extensively. For some people, talking things out helps them process their feelings, and having someone listen without offering advice or solutions might validate their experience.

Ask your partner what they need. There is a common assumption that people in partnerships should naturally comprehend and anticipate their partner's wants. In truth, no one can read minds, and even the most smart and intuitive partners occasionally require guidance. If your partner is experiencing infertility, don't be scared to ask them what they need or what sort of support they want. Adapt your lifestyle with them. When someone is undergoing fertility treatment, such as IVF, they are frequently restricted from consuming alcohol and tobacco.

If possible, adjusting your lifestyle to match theirs can be affirming and a tangible method to express your support. If they are unable to drink, avoid doing so around them. Even if your partner does not express a need for this form of support, offering to abstain with them demonstrates participation and investment in your family's journey. Be involved.

Fertility treatment can be time-consuming, with many checkups, check-ins, and tracking. Being physically present during your partner's appointments and actively participating in their experience can help to relieve some of their stress.

During doctor's visits, you can take notes or remind your partner of things they intended to ask. If possible, acquaint yourself with the language used when discussing treatment so that your spouse can refer to words without explanation.

Logistics Support: Sperm analysis Male infertility accounts for 20-30% of fertility issues, while women are frequently blamed for infertility. A semen analysis is a concrete technique for guys whose female partners are undergoing reproductive treatment to express support while ruling out any other variables. A semen analysis will assess semen volume and pH, as well as sperm concentration, morphology, and motility, all of which might influence the likelihood of sperm fertilizing the egg.

Blood Test. Similarly to sperm testing, blood testing allows men to easily rule out any potential causes of infertility. Follicle-stimulating hormone (FSH) testing in men can evaluate sperm count while luteinizing hormone (LH) testing helps guarantee that testosterone production is stimulated.

Prolactin and androgen tests are also used to diagnose erectile dysfunction or low libido. Keep them on track. When undergoing fertility treatment, there are usually several drugs, supplements, procedures, and appointments to handle.

Helping your spouse keep track of all these moving elements demonstrates vital support and allows them to prioritize self-care, which is especially crucial during treatment.

CHAPTER 10

Keeping A Good Attitude And Practical Ideas For Managing Treatment

Importance of a Positive Attitude A good attitude can have a huge impact on your reproductive journey, boosting emotional resilience and overall well-being. While remaining positive does not ensure success, it does aid in coping with problems, making informed decisions, and enhancing quality of life while in treatment.

Here's How To Cultivate A Good Mindset And Practical Ideas For Managing Fertility Treatment:

Fostering A Positive Attitude Focus On What You Can Control. Take Charge: Take an active role in your treatment strategy. This can include following medical recommendations, monitoring ovulation, and adopting lifestyle adjustments.

Set realistic goals. Divide the journey into tiny, doable steps. Celebrate little successes, such as finishing a treatment cycle or changing your lifestyle choices.

Practice Gratitude. Daily Reflections: Keep a thankfulness diary to record great experiences, supportive encounters, and everything that made you happy throughout the day.

Focus On The Present: Instead of focusing entirely on the end objective, try to embrace the positive aspects of your current circumstances.

Develop A Support System. Share your emotions and experiences with close friends and family members who can offer emotional support.

Join Supporting Groups: Engage in local or online networks of people going through similar circumstances. Sharing tales and suggestions may be both comforting and motivating.

Stay Informed But Balanced. Educate Yourself: Understanding your treatment options and the fertility process might make you feel less anxious and more in control. Avoid information overload by balancing it with activities that help you rest and unwind. Too much knowledge might cause tension.

Engage In Positive Visualization Imagine Success: Take a few minutes each day to envision happy outcomes, such as a successful therapy or holding your baby. This can instill optimism and alleviate tension.

Affirmations: Use positive affirmations to help you stay hopeful and resilient. Statements such as "I am doing everything I can" can be motivating.

Practical Strategies For Managing Treatment

Prepare Your Treatment Plan. Create A Schedule: Maintain a thorough calendar with all appointments, prescription regimes, and significant dates. This aids in staying organized and eliminates the possibility of missing important steps.

Prepare Questions. Before your appointments, write down any questions or concerns you want to discuss with your healthcare professional. This helps you get the most out of your consultations. Communicate with your healthcare team.

Establish a positive rapport with your doctors and nurses. Clear and honest communication might make you feel more supported and involved in your treatment.

Seek Clarifications: Do not be afraid to ask for clarifications about treatment options, procedures, and potential adverse effects. Understanding your treatment can help alleviate anxiety.

Monitor Your Health Track Symptoms: Keep track of your physical and emotional symptoms throughout treatment. This information can help your healthcare practitioner change your treatment plan.

Stay Active: Moderate exercise can help enhance physical health and reduce stress. Walking, swimming, and yoga are all healthy activities. Manage medications and supplements.

Set Reminders: Use alarms or apps to remind you to take your meds and supplements on schedule. Treatment effectiveness relies heavily on consistency.

Organize Supplies: Keep all medications, vitamins, and injectable supplies in a specific location to eliminate last-minute searches.

Plan For Financial Management. Understand Costs: Talk to your clinic about treatment costs and, if necessary, look into insurance coverage. Understanding the money component can help you avoid unforeseen stress.

Budgeting: Make a budget that covers all treatment-related charges and look into financial help, grants, or payment plans provided by clinics. Prioritize self-care.

Rest And Relax: Get enough sleep and practice relaxing techniques like deep breathing, meditation, or hobbies you love.

Nutrition: Eat a balanced diet high in nutrients that promote reproductive health. Consult a dietitian if you need to alter your diet for fertility. Seek emotional support.

Counseling: Seek treatment from an infertility therapist to manage stress, worry, and any marital pressure. Allow yourself to experience and express a variety of emotions. Bottled-up emotions can lead to greater tension and worry.

Stay Flexible. Adaptability: Be prepared to adjust your treatment approach based on how your body responds. Flexibility can help you deal with unanticipated obstacles.

Resilience: Build resilience by focusing on your strengths and the support system around you. Building resilience can help you recover from setbacks.

Maintaining a positive attitude and managing therapy correctly can dramatically improve your fertility experience. You may face obstacles with greater resilience and hope if you focus on what you can control, keep informed, organize your treatment plan, and seek help. Remember that every step, no matter how tiny, gets you closer to your objective, and your efforts are valuable.

CHAPTER 11

Success Stories

Here are a few success stories that highlight the achievements and joys felt by couples on their reproductive journeys:

Joy And Samuel's Miracle Babies

Joy and Samuel were depressed and despairing after years of unsuccessful attempts to conceive. They opted to consult a reproductive doctor, who diagnosed Joy with polycystic ovarian syndrome (PCOS). Joy and Samuel finally had their long-awaited baby daughter after combining medicine, lifestyle adjustments, and IVF. Their journey was fraught with ups and downs, but their persistent perseverance and the encouragement of their loved ones led to their eventual achievement.

Ruth And John's Journey To Parenthood

Ruth and John had always wanted to start a family together, but after several losses and unsuccessful reproductive treatments, they began to lose hope.

Despite the hurdles, they refused to give up on their dream. They investigated various treatment options under the supervision of their reproductive clinic before achieving success with a mix of IVF and genetic screening. Ruth and John are now proud parents of twins, a boy and a girl, and their experience has taught them the value of resilience and endurance.

Ella And Amos's Unexpected Blessing

Ella and Amos had accepted that they might never have their children. After years of fruitless reproductive treatments, they chose to focus on creating a happy life as a couple. However, Ella unexpectedly realized she was pregnant. Despite the chances, their little miracle arrived alive and well, bringing immeasurable joy and appreciation into their lives.

These success stories serve as reminders that, while the route to motherhood may be difficult, with perseverance, support, and an optimistic attitude, dreams may be realized. Each trip is unique, but the end outcome always demonstrates the human spirit's strength and endurance.

Conclusion

As we conclude "How to Win the Fertility Battle: Navigating the Path to Parenthood," I'd like to leave you with a message of hope, perseverance, and unshakable persistence.

Throughout this book, we've looked at the obstacles and successes of the fertility journey, learning vital lessons along the way. Remember that you are not alone if you have gone through infertility. Your journey is unique, but many others understand the highs and lows you experience.

You can negotiate the uncertainties of infertility with fortitude and courage by accepting assistance from loved ones, receiving advice from healthcare specialists, and having a good attitude. While the path to motherhood is fraught with challenges, it is also paved with moments of joy, perseverance, and deep love.

Whether you conceive naturally, through fertility treatments, or alternate avenues such as adoption or surrogacy, remember that the love you have to give as a parent is immeasurable.

As you shut the last pages of this book, may you carry with you the wisdom, encouragement, and inspiration contained inside its pages.

May you approach each day with hope and resolve. And may your parenting journey be filled with the gifts of love, joy, and fresh starts.

Best wishes for your reproductive journey and beyond.

www.ingramcontent.com/pod-product-compliance
Lightning Source LLC
Chambersburg PA
CBHW050815250726
48653CB00006B/2245